The Library of Sexual Health™

ENDOMETRIOSIS

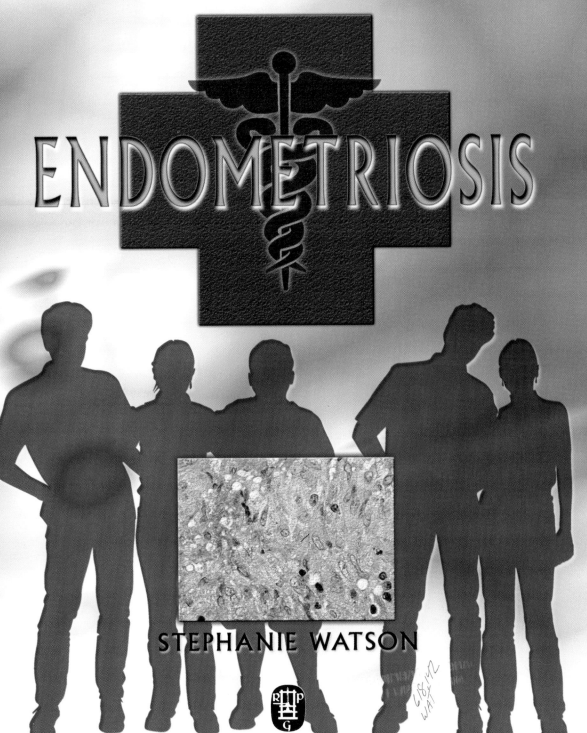

STEPHANIE WATSON

The Rosen Publishing Group, Inc., New York

To my supportive husband, Ken, and my wonderful little boy, Jake

Published in 2007 by The Rosen Publishing Group, Inc.
29 East 21st Street, New York, NY 10010

Library of Congress Cataloging-in-Publication Data

Watson, Stephanie, 1969–
Endometriosis/Stephanie Watson.—1st ed.
    p. cm.—(The library of sexual health)
Includes bibliographical references and index.
ISBN-13: 978-1-4042-0904-6
ISBN-10: 1-4042-0904-2 (library binding)
1. Endometriosis—Juvenile literature. I. Title. II. Series.
RG483.E53W38 2007
618.1—dc22

                                                    2006002103

Manufactured in the United States of America

CONTENTS

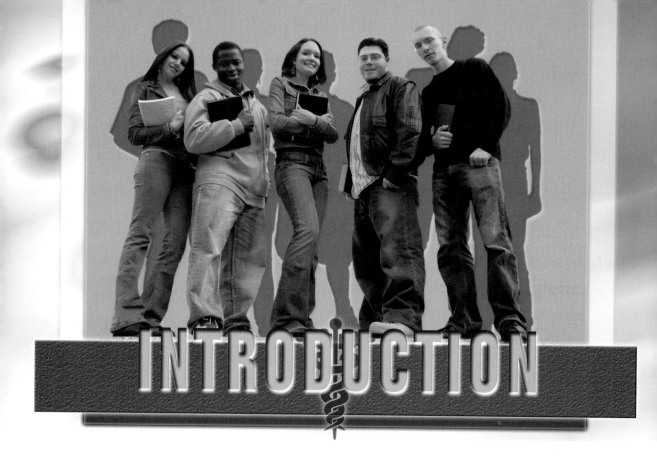

INTRODUCTION

E ndometriosis . . . it's a mysterious condition with a strange-sounding name. Millions of women have it, but many don't know they do.

What is endometriosis? What does it do to the body? And what should you do if you think you have it?

Endometriosis involves the period, or menstruation. Getting your first period, known as menarche, is one of the most important times in your life. It means that you are beginning your menstrual cycle and are becoming a woman. Some girls look forward to their first period. Others find that getting their periods is a bit annoying or embarrassing, but they get used to it after a while.

But some girls worry about getting their periods because they can be inconvenient or even painful. It's different for everybody. Some girls have cramps that are not too painful. Others experience very painful cramps when they get their periods. Intense cramps during periods can be a sign of endometriosis. This disease happens when tissue similar to the inside lining of the uterus ends up in other parts of the body. Endometriosis affects at least 5.5 million women in North America, according to the National Institutes of Health (NIH). The disease can affect girls and women from ages eight to eighty.

Although no one is really sure exactly how many teenage girls get endometriosis, most women who have the condition say it started for them soon after they got their first period. Many girls don't get diagnosed because they don't understand what they're feeling or they're too embarrassed or afraid to tell anyone about it.

Doctors don't know for sure what causes endometriosis. It's hard to diagnose and difficult to treat. Some doctors say that feeling *discomfort* is just part of getting a period. But endometriosis is a real medical condition.

If you have endometriosis, it can get in the way of doing things you enjoy. You may have to skip important events. You may be absent from school often and have to catch up on homework. You may miss soccer, ballet, music lessons, and other activities.

Having endometriosis can present challenges. If you have it, you may be afraid to tell your family and friends. It's hard to explain a disease that most people know little about. You may be ashamed of having endometriosis because it involves your reproductive organs. Or you may think that having it is your fault. In reality, there is no way you could have prevented it. And there is no need to feel ashamed. And, remember, if you do have endometriosis, there are places to get help and ways to feel better.

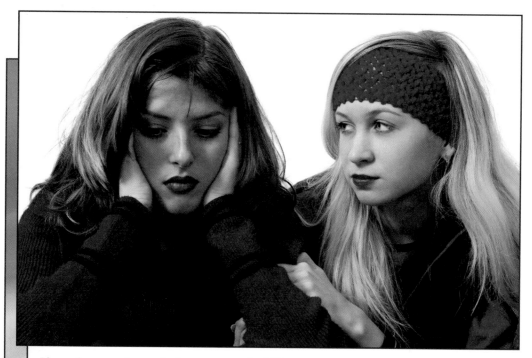

If you have endometriosis, you may feel like you can't tell anyone. It's often hard to explain the disease to family and friends who don't understand what it's all about.

This book will explain how the female reproductive organs work. It will show you how people might get endometriosis. It will explain how you can find out if you have it. You will learn what the symptoms are and where to go for help. You'll also find out about new treatments.

You will learn that millions of women have endometriosis. And you will see that there is no reason to be ashamed. There is also no reason to live in pain when treatments are available. By learning all you can about this disease, you will be able to get help or give support to a friend who has endometriosis.

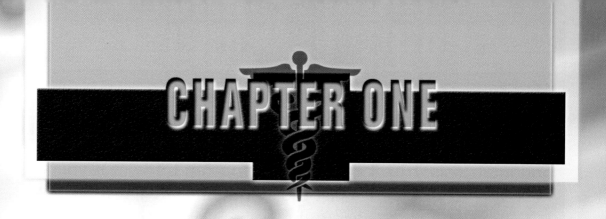

CHAPTER ONE

What Is Endometriosis?

This strange-sounding name is for a disease many people know little about. What does "endometriosis" mean? How does someone get it? And what happens to you if you do get it?

Endometriosis gets its name from the endometrium, the tissue that lines the uterus. When tissue like the tissue that lines the uterus grows in places where it doesn't belong, it is endometriosis.

In people with endometriosis, the tissue grows around the ovaries, uterus, fallopian tubes, or on the pelvic wall. It can also grow on the bladder, intestines, rectum, and scars in the abdomen from surgeries. In very rare cases, this tissue can be found as far away from the uterus as the lungs, arms and thighs, or head. The misplaced tissue builds up and forms growths. These growths have many names, including lesions, nodules, or implants. We'll call them lesions.

Even though the lesions are in other parts of the body, they still act somewhat like tissue in the uterus.

Every month, hormones tell the uterine lining to build up and then shed. When the tissue sheds from the uterus, it leaves the body through menstruation.

Hormones also tell endometriosis tissue in other parts of the body to build up and then shed. When the tissue is in the wrong place, it has no way to exit the body. It builds up and makes chemicals that irritate nearby tissue. This causes swelling, pain, and sometimes scarring in the area around the tissue.

ENDOMETRIOSIS AND YOUR BODY

Endometriosis occurs when tissue similar to the endometrium, the layer of tissue that lines the uterus, grows in other parts of the body. To understand it, you have to know a little about how the female body works.

The Female Reproductive System

The female reproductive system is made up of two parts: external genitals and internal organs. On the

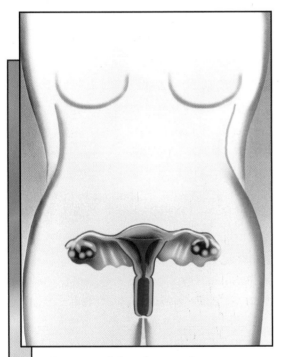

The internal female reproductive organs include the ovaries, uterus, and cervix. The two ovaries make female hormones and contain sacs in which the eggs form. The uterus is the pear-shaped organ that opens into the vagina through the cervix.

Jenna's Story

Jenna was fourteen years old when she had her first period. She was scared, but a little excited, too. She felt like she was finally an adult. But when she got her second period, the pain hit. It was so strong that she couldn't stand up. She had to lie in bed for hours at a time.

Her mother told her that having painful cramps was normal during menstruation. When Jenna felt the pain during gym class, her gym teacher also told her that experiencing pain was normal. Even some of her friends told her it was nothing to worry about.

But Jenna was in pain every month for almost a year. She missed a few days of school each month. She also missed horseback riding and violin lessons. Jenna couldn't attend her friend Aurelia's "sweet sixteen" party.

Jenna's mother finally took her to a gynecologist. This is a special doctor for women. The doctor told her she just had painful periods. He gave her a prescription pain reliever to relax her muscles and ease the discomfort and aching. But the pain didn't go away.

One day, Jenna was doing research on the Web for a school paper for biology class. When she looked up her symptoms, she saw the word "endometriosis." Jenna wondered if she might have endometriosis, so she went back to her doctor for an examination. He carefully checked her again and used a procedure called ultrasound to look inside her body.

The doctor told Jenna that she probably did have endometriosis and that she needed to undergo a procedure called laparoscopy. She had to go to the hospital and was given anesthetics, which made her fall asleep. The doctor filled Jenna's abdomen with a gas. Then he used a thin, lighted tube to look inside her body. While he was performing the laparoscopy, he used a laser to remove some of the disease that was causing Jenna's pain.

When Jenna woke up, the doctor told her that she definitely had endometriosis. There is no cure for it, he said. The doctor prescribed special pills for Jenna to take. The pills had hormones in them. He wanted to see if they would make her feel better so he wouldn't have to do more surgery.

Jenna began taking the pills and they stopped her period. Her pain faded. Soon, she was able to go to school full-time and resume her usual activities. Jenna will possibly never be cured of endometriosis, but by managing her pain and taking responsibility for her own health and well-being, she can enjoy a very active and productive life.

outside of the body are the vulva and vagina. "Vulva" is a word for all the outer genital organs. The vagina is the canal that leads from the outside of the body to the cervix inside. It is where menstrual fluid comes out during a period. It is also where a baby would come out during childbirth.

Inside a woman's body are the main structures of the female reproductive system. These structures are

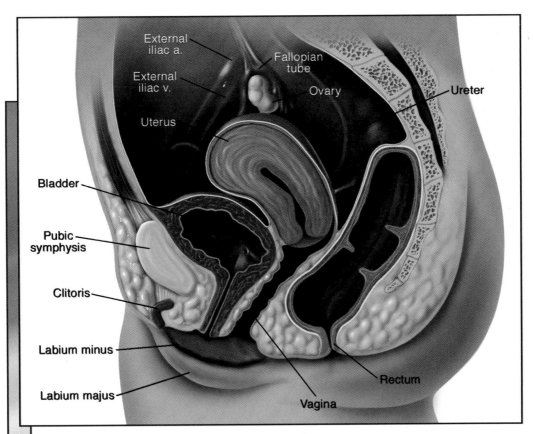

The vulva and vagina are the external female reproductive organs. The vulva includes the labia, clitoris, and opening to the vagina. The vagina is the canal that leads into the cervix.

the ovaries, fallopian tubes, uterus, and cervix. Let's consider each of these parts:

- **Ovaries.** These are the two female sex glands. They have sacs in which eggs, called ova, form. They also make female hormones.
- **Fallopian tubes.** These are the tubes through which an egg passes to be fertilized by sperm.
- **Uterus.** This is the pear-shaped organ that will hold the fetus during pregnancy. Tissue similar to the inside lining of the uterus is involved in endometriosis.
- **Cervix.** This is the lower part of the uterus that extends down into the top of the vagina.

The female reproductive system gets a woman's body ready to help an embryo grow.

YOUR PERIOD

If you have already started your period, you know that you bleed every month. What causes that bleeding? A period is all about getting an egg ready to be fertilized.

Every month, your body releases hormones that tell an egg to develop in your ovary. The entire cycle of the egg maturing and being released from the body is called the menstrual cycle. At around the middle of the cycle, hormone levels surge. The increase in hormones causes the ovary to release a mature egg. It's a process called ovulation.

The released egg moves through one of the fallopian tubes and into the uterus. It takes about four or five days for the egg to get there. If a woman has had sexual intercourse recently, sperm might be present along the route. In that case, the egg may be fertilized. The woman could get pregnant.

During the menstrual cycle, the uterus becomes thick with blood vessels and endometrial tissue. These will nourish the egg if it is fertilized. If you don't get pregnant, you no longer need the tissue. Hormones tell the uterus

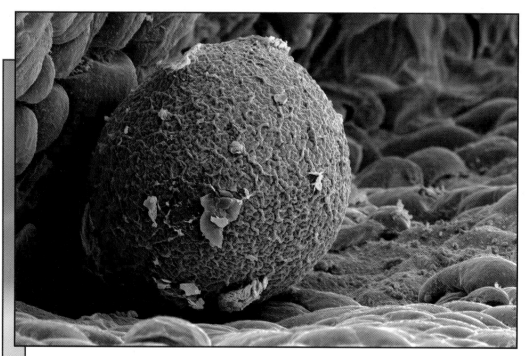

This is an egg that has been fertilized by a man's sperm. The fertilized egg will travel down the fallopian tube to implant in the uterus, which will house and nourish the growing fetus.

to shed it. The tissue leaves your body, along with blood and mucus, through the vagina. This is how you have your period. Shedding these materials gets your body ready for the new menstrual cycle. However, if you have endometriosis, the lesions outside your uterus bleed, too, during your period. Blood or tissue from endometriosis that is shed during this process can't leave your body. This results in inflammation and pain, and scar tissue may develop. Scar tissue can also cause more inflammation and pain.

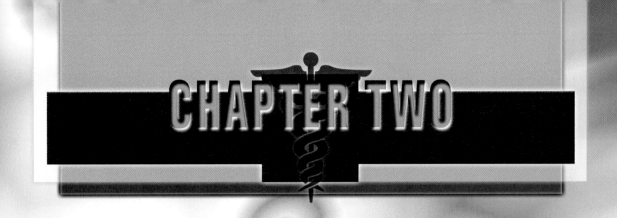

CHAPTER TWO

Mysterious Condition

Medicine today can do amazing things. It can replace parts of the body that are damaged by injury or disease. It can cure diseases that were once impossible to treat. But as modern as medicine is, it can't cure endometriosis yet. Doctors don't know exactly what causes this disease. They do have a few ideas about some causes, though, and about some factors that are believed to influence the development of the disease.

DISCOVERING ENDOMETRIOSIS

Doctors have known about endometriosis for many years. The first person to describe the disease as we know it today was an Austrian doctor named Karl von Rokitansky (1804–1878), in 1860. New York surgeon John Sampson (1873–1946) saw a possible cause of endometriosis. In the 1920s, he was operating on a woman when he saw endo- metrial tissue in the wrong part of her body. He came up with the idea that the tissue flows back through the

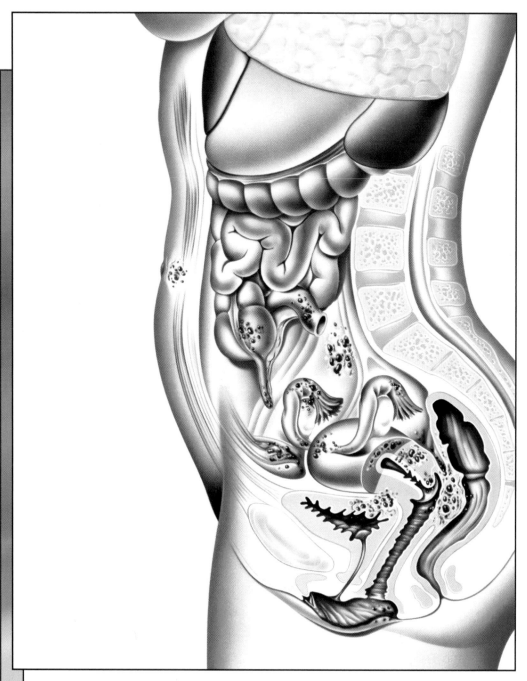

Endometriosis occurs when tissue similar to the tissue normally lining the uterus grows in other parts of the body. The places in which endometriosis tissue often grows are shown in blue. They include *(from top to bottom)*: the abdomen, intestines, fallopian tubes, ovaries, appendix, uterus, peritoneum (lining of the abdomen), cervix, rectum, bladder, and vulva.

fallopian tubes during a woman's period. Sampson believed that tissue could become implanted in other places in the body.

Many people have different ideas about the causes. Some doctors follow Sampson's theory that this backup of tissue leads to endometriosis. They think that some of the tissue a woman sheds during her period backs up through the fallopian tubes and grows in other places.

Many women have this backup of tissue, but not all have endometriosis. So why don't all of them get it? An individual's immune system may be a factor. The immune system keeps a person healthy by fighting off foreign invaders. These invaders may be bacteria and other germs from outside an individual's body. They may also be substances the body makes that go someplace by mistake. A woman who has endometriosis has an immune system that doesn't treat misplaced tissue as foreign. The immune system lets the tissue grow in the wrong place. This woman's body may even help it grow.

Another way that endometriosis tissue could travel is through tubes called lymph vessels or through blood vessels. The tissue then implants itself wherever it ends up. Joseph Halban (1890–1937) came up with this theory in the 1920s. His idea might explain how endometriosis can occur as far as the bladder or lungs.

A doctor named R. Meyer had another idea in 1919. He thought that the problem starts before a girl is even born. When sperm and egg merge to form an embryo, that embryo contains all the cells needed to grow every organ and tissue in the baby's body. Certain cells develop into organs and tissues, such as a heart or kidneys. Meyer said that cells in the wrong part of the embryo (such as in the ovaries) change into endometrial tissue by mistake and then grow there.

Some doctors think that chemicals called dioxins and PCBs (polychlorinated biphenyls) may have something to do with endometriosis. They are two very toxic chemical compounds.

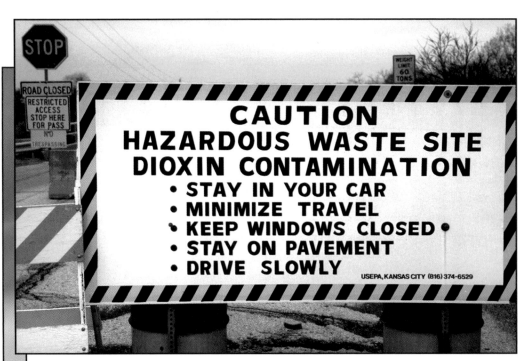

Some people believe that exposure to toxic chemicals in the environment can lead to endometriosis. Dioxins and PCBs are two possible culprits.

Dioxins are the by-products of manufacturing processes, such as the smelting of metals, the making of plastics, and the bleaching of paper pulp. Once they are released into the environment or get into our bodies, dioxins can stay there for a long time, on average about fourteen years, since they build up in body fats and are chemically stable.

PCBs are mixtures of chemicals that were once used as coolants and lubricants in transformers and other electrical equipment. The manufacture of PCBs stopped in 1977, but products made before that year, such as electrical devices and fluorescent lights, can still contain them. Exposure to dioxins and PCBs may damage a person's immune and reproductive systems.

These are just ideas, or theories, about endometriosis. No one knows for sure what causes it. More than one reason may be involved.

COULD I GET ENDOMETRIOSIS?

There is no way to know for sure who will get endometriosis. There are certain similarities in people who have it. Most people who are diagnosed with endometriosis are between the ages of twenty and forty. But it's very common to find endometriosis in teens. Girls as young as eight or nine have it, and women as old as sixty or seventy can still have it. If you have the disease, you may not start having symptoms of endometriosis until you have started menstruation. Symptoms may start with gastrointestinal discomfort.

Myths and Facts

MYTH: It is normal to have severe pain during your period.
FACT: Periods can cause cramps, but they should never be more than a mild sensation, not painful.

MYTH: Very young girls don't get endometriosis.
FACT: Endometriosis can start as young as age eight or nine, even before the first period.

MYTH: Surgery will cure endometriosis.
FACT: There is no cure, but surgery can ease the symptoms.

MYTH: You have to put up with the pain of endometriosis.
FACT: There are treatments for endometriosis. You don't have to suffer from pain.

You are more likely to get endometriosis if your mother or sister has it. There may be one or more changes to genes that are passed down through families. Doctors haven't found those genetic changes yet, though. Families also share environments, and that may contribute to the shared risk. You also may be more at risk if your uterus is tipped forward or backward, or if you have a narrow or missing cervix.

WHAT CAN I DO TO PREVENT ENDOMETRIOSIS?

Some diseases can be prevented. You can avoid getting a sexually transmitted disease (STD), such as chlamydia, by using a condom during sexual intercourse. You can prevent the mumps by getting a vaccine for it. But you may not be able to completely prevent endometriosis because no one knows what causes it yet.

There are things you can do to protect yourself, though. Take care of your body. Eat a healthy diet with reduced amounts of sugar, salt, and processed foods. Good nutrition will affect your physical and emotional health. Get plenty of exercise as well.

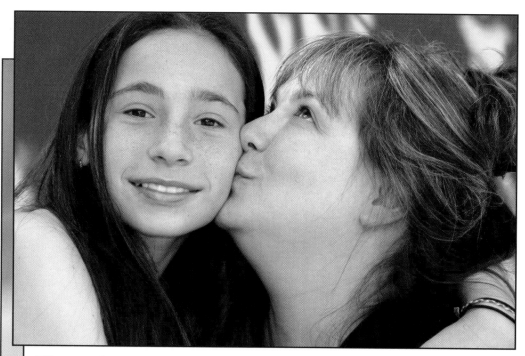

When you have endometriosis, it's important to remember that your disease is not your fault. Know that you can get help and support from friends, family, doctors, and support groups.

If you have pain or other symptoms, see a doctor who specializes in endometriosis. There are several treatment options available, and together with your parents and your doctor, you can determine what your goals are in managing and treating your endometriosis.

Remember that endometriosis is not your fault. The important thing is to get it diagnosed and treated as early as possible.

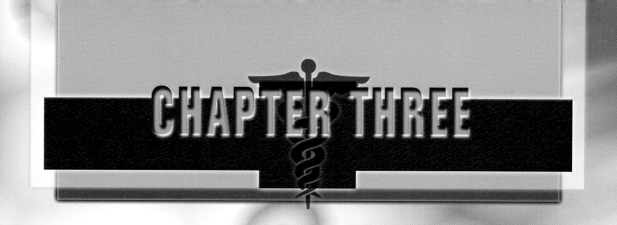

CHAPTER THREE

Knowing for Sure

You may have endometriosis if you have some of these symptoms:

- **Pain.** This is the main symptom of endometriosis. The lesions cause swelling that pushes on other tissues, irritating them. They also release substances that are similar to hormones and that cause pain. These substances are called prostaglandins. The pain can feel like cramps in your abdomen. Or, you might feel it in your back, pelvis, or bladder. It might hurt when you urinate or have a bowel movement. Or sexual intercourse might hurt. It depends on where the lesions are located and other factors. The pain can be so strong that you can't get out of bed during your period. It can last through your whole period. Some women with endometriosis have no pain, though. Strangely enough, the amount of pain you feel has nothing to do with the size or number of the lesions. Small lesions may cause more pain than big lesions in some people.

- **Irregular bleeding.** Your periods may be heavier than normal. Or, you may bleed or spot between periods.
- **Intestinal problems.** You may not be able to have a bowel movement. Or, you may go to the bathroom too often and have loose stools. You may also feel bloated, have pain during bowel movements, or have bleeding from the rectal area. Lesions in your intestines may also make you feel nauseated or make you vomit.

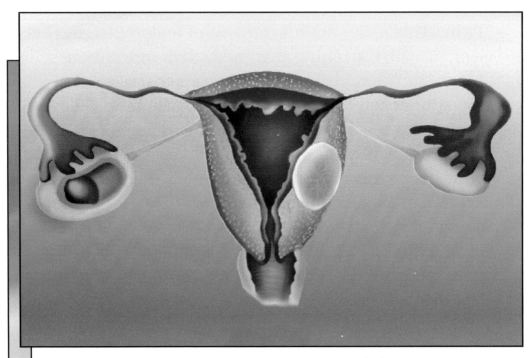

An ovarian cyst (shown here at the left) is a small growth that forms on your ovary. Sometimes that growth can break open and leak fluid. A fibroma (seen here in the uterine wall), also called fibroid, is a non-cancerous tumor.

- **Urinary problems.** You may have pain when you urinate or have trouble urinating if the lesions are on your bladder.
- **Ovarian cysts.** On your ovary, you may get a small growth called a cyst. This growth can break and leak fluid. These cysts are sometimes called chocolate cysts, since the fluid inside contains old, brown blood.

Not everyone with endometriosis will have these symptoms. Some people feel fine, while others hurt all the time. Also, many other conditions can cause these same symptoms. Cysts, pregnancy, pelvic inflammatory disease, irritable bowel syndrome, and appendicitis can all have the same symptoms. That's why it's important to see a specialized doctor if you're feeling any of these things.

THE RISK OF INFERTILITY

One of the risks with endometriosis is not being able to have children. This is called infertility. About 30 to 40 percent of women with endometriosis are infertile, according to research studies. Endometriosis tissue makes it difficult for a woman to have a baby because it affects her reproductive organs. The tissue can block the fallopian tubes so the eggs can't go down them to the uterus. It also can affect the lining of the uterus so that an embryo can't implant and grow.

Some women don't find out that they can't get pregnant until they try to have a baby. When a woman tries to have a baby for a year without using a condom or other contraception and she can't get pregnant, she is said to be infertile.

Some women with endometriosis can get pregnant, but they have trouble carrying the baby to full term. Endometriosis increases the risk for ectopic pregnancy. This is when the embryo grows outside the uterus. It may even grow in the fallopian tubes. This is dangerous because the space is too small for the baby to grow. A woman who has this problem may need surgery to stop the pregnancy before it threatens her life.

ENDOMETRIOSIS AND CANCER

Endometriosis is not cancer. Cancer occurs when cells grow and divide out of control. They keep growing until they form lumps called tumors. Cancer cells can spread to other organs and damage them. If cancer is caught early, before it has a chance to spread to other organs or to damage them, people can be treated and they can survive their cancer. Cells in endometriosis tissue are not the same as cancer cells, but they can also spread in the body. They can damage organs, including the ovaries, bladder, and bowel. But even though you may feel a lot of pain, people don't usually die from endometriosis.

If you have endometriosis, some research shows that it could increase your risk for having certain types of cancer. One study found that endometriosis increased a woman's risk of getting ovarian cancer by just under a half, endocrine cancer by about a third, non-Hodgkin's lymphoma by about a quarter, and brain cancers by about a fifth. Remember, though, that having an increased risk does not mean that you will get cancer.

No one knows why women with endometriosis have a greater risk of developing cancer. It may be because the immune system does not work like it should.

SEEING YOUR DOCTOR FOR THE FIRST TIME

Going to a gynecologist for the first time can be scary. You may not know what to expect. You may be ashamed to talk about your symptoms. If this is true, you are not alone. Many women wait for as long as ten years before getting diagnosed because they don't want to tell their doctors. Others have to visit many doctors before getting the right diagnosis.

If you have any of the symptoms, see a gynecologist. On your first visit, the doctor will look at your medical history. She will also ask about your family medical history. Knowing if your mother or sister has endometriosis can make it easier for her to diagnose you. She'll ask you what symptoms you've been having, especially pain. She may ask you to rate your pain on a scale of one to ten, where one is very mild pain and ten is very severe pain.

It may help if you keep a diary of your pain before your doctor's visit. In this diary, you write down every time you have endometriosis pain. You also write what you were doing when the pain hit, and what you did to ease the pain. Your diary may look something like this:

Date	Activity	Pain Level	Pain Location	How Long It Lasted	Action Taken
Dec. 10	Jogging	10	Abdomen	1 hour	Stopped jogging and felt better.
Dec. 10	Watching television	3	Abdomen	2 hours	Took Tylenol and felt better.
Dec. 11	At school	6	Lower back	½ hour	Rested in the nurse's office and felt better.

Keeping a diary can help you answer your doctor's questions. These are some of the questions she might ask:

- When did your pain start?
- Where is the pain located?
- What does it feel like (burning, achy, stabbing, etc.)?
- How strong is the pain (on a scale of one to ten)?

- How often do you feel the pain?
- When does it happen (for example, when you're exercising)?
- How long does the pain last?
- Do you have any bloating or swelling in your abdomen?
- Do you have pain while urinating or having bowel movements?

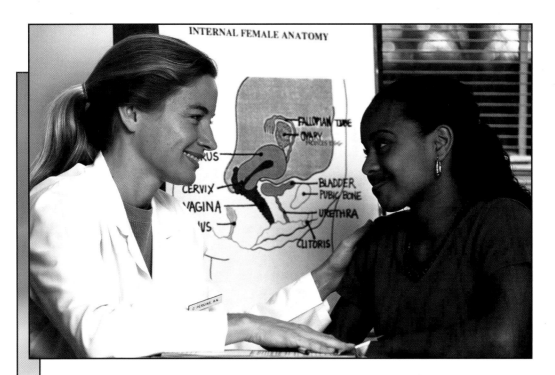

To make a diagnosis of your health condition, the doctor will ask you many questions about your disease. It will be easier for you to answer her questions if you keep a diary of your symptoms before your visit.

- Are you sexually active? If so, do you feel pain during or after sex?
- Do you have any allergies? Do you have asthma or eczema?

If your doctor suspects that you have endometriosis, she will examine you to feel for any lesions in your pelvic area. This is called a pelvic exam. You may be scared if you have never had this kind of exam before. You may be embarrassed. If you are too scared or embarrassed, ask your doctor if you can have other tests first.

TESTS FOR ENDOMETRIOSIS

Sometimes doctors can feel lesions during a pelvic exam. The doctor may also send you for a test that takes a picture of the inside of your body through your abdomen. The test may use one of a few different types of machines to take this picture. An ultrasound uses sound waves to take the picture. Magnetic resonance imaging (MRI) uses magnets and radio waves to take the picture. Computed tomography (CT) scans take X-ray pictures from many different angles. A computer combines those images to show a more complete picture of the body. These tests are useful, but they can't tell for sure whether you have endometriosis.

If your doctor still suspects that you have endometriosis, she may give you medicine to ease your pain. If the medicine doesn't help, your doctor may want you to have a surgical procedure called laparoscopy. This is the

only way to know for certain if you have endometriosis.
Your doctor needs to diagnose endometriosis before
treating it.

Laparoscopy isn't like regular surgery, because the
incisions, or cuts, are much smaller. A doctor called an
anesthesiologist will put you to sleep with drugs called
general anesthetics so you won't feel pain during the
surgery. The doctor will first put carbon dioxide gas in
your abdomen to make it bigger. This will help her see your
ovaries, fallopian tubes, uterus, and other organs to look

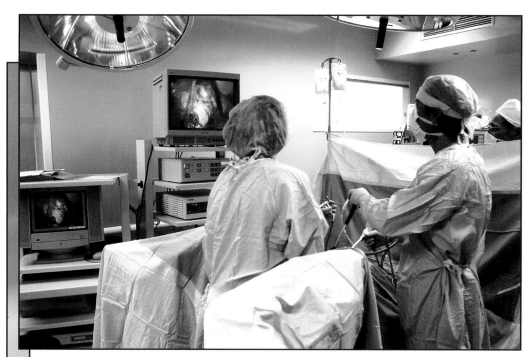

If medicine alone isn't enough to relieve your pain, your doctor may perform a type
of surgery called laparoscopy. During this procedure, the doctor will use a thin,
lighted scope to look for endometriosis inside your body and remove it.

for endometrial lesions. Then, the doctor will make a very small incision near your belly button.

A thin tube called an endoscope will go inside your body through one cut. This scope will help the doctor see your organs and find endometriosis. The scope has a tiny camera on it that takes images of the inside of your body. The doctor can see those images on a video monitor connected to the scope or right through the scope.

If you do have endometriosis, the doctor can remove a piece of tissue by making another cut and inserting a laser or other surgical instrument through it. The tissue will be sent to a lab, where someone will look at it under a microscope to see what kinds of cells are there and to make sure it isn't cancer. It probably won't be cancer, but doctors always want to make sure. The tissue sample is called a biopsy. During the surgery, your doctor may also remove some of the endometriosis tissue to ease your pain. After your surgery, you should be able to go home. You may have a very small scar at the site of each incision.

STAGES OF ENDOMETRIOSIS

Surgery helps the doctor find out if you have endometriosis. It also helps the doctor determine what stage of the disease you have. Endometriosis has been classified into four stages by the American Society for Reproductive Medicine (ASRM), formerly known as the American Fertility Society. The stages are based on the size, location, and number of lesions. The higher the stage, the more serious the endometriosis. But the pain you are feeling may have nothing to do with your stage. It's possible to have a lot of pain, even in stage 1.

These are the four stages for endometriosis:

- **Stage 1–Minimal.** The lesions are only in the abdomen and one ovary. The lesions aren't very deep.
- **Stage 2–Mild.** The lesions are in the abdomen and both ovaries. They may or may not be deep.
- **Stage 3–Moderate.** The lesions are in the abdomen, both ovaries, and both fallopian tubes.
- **Stage 4–Severe.** The lesions may be in other parts of the body.

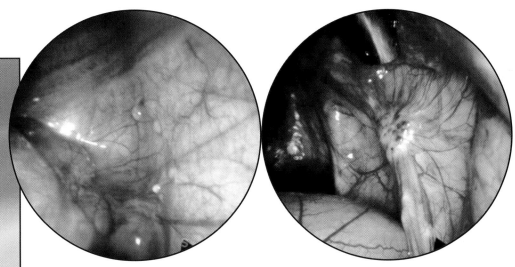

This is what endometriosis looks like when a doctor examines it through a laparo-scope. The photograph at the left shows a teenager's lesions; the one at the right shows lesions in a thirty-five-year-old.

Even though your doctor may identify the stage of your condition, that doesn't describe how you are feeling. You may have very few lesions, but you hurt all the time. Or, you may have a lot of lesions but feel very good. Together with you and your parents, your doctor can help find the right treatment for you based on both the stage of endometriosis and how you feel.

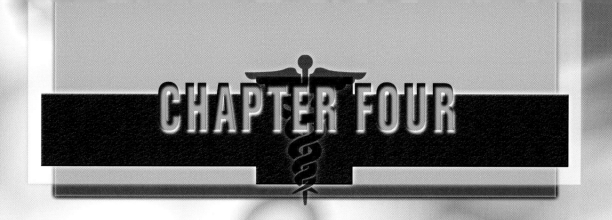

CHAPTER FOUR

Treating Endometriosis

T here is no cure for endometriosis. There are treatments, though, that can ease your pain and reduce your other symptoms. Medicine and surgery are the two most common types of treatment. They work by shrinking the lesions. Which treatment you and your parents decide to follow with your doctor may depend on your age, health, and how bad your symptoms are. The following are some of the different endometriosis treatments that are available to you.

PAIN MEDICATIONS

The main symptom of endometriosis is pain. Your doctor may give you medicine to help you hurt less. You may take NSAIDs (nonsteroidal anti-inflammatory drugs). These pills decrease swelling and pain. You may get an NSAID such as Aleve, Naprosyn, Motrin, or Advil. You can buy many of these NSAIDs right off the shelf at your local supermarket or drugstore. Other medicine requires a prescription from your doctor. All of these drugs work about the same. They work best for mild pain. NSAIDs are generally safe, but they can cause stomach problems. Always take them with food.

Aspirin and acetaminophen (such as Tylenol) are two other types of pain relievers. They also can cause upset stomach.

If your pain is really severe, you may need stronger drugs. These can give you greater relief, but they can

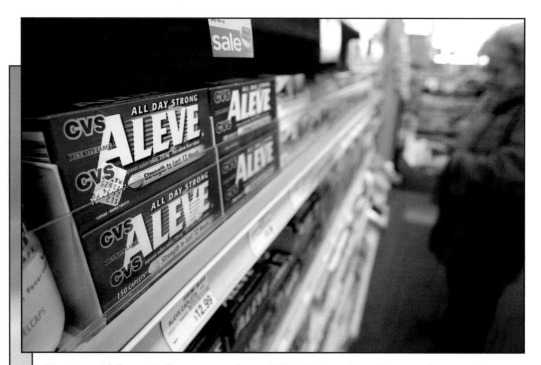

Non-steroidal anti-inflammatory drugs (NSAIDs) such as Aleve reduce swelling and ease the pain of endometriosis. You can buy these types of medicine in your local supermarket or drugstore without a prescription.

have some pretty bad side effects. Narcotics, such as morphine and codeine, act on the brain and spinal cord. They dull the feeling of pain. But they can make you feel tired and confused. You may have to get off these drugs gradually once your pain eases.

HORMONE DRUGS

Hormones control the menstrual cycle. Endometriosis pain usually occurs before or during your period, but it can sometimes occur in the middle of the cycle (ovulation). Some drugs slow down or stop your period to relieve the pain. They work on the hormones that control ovulation and menstruation. You take hormone drugs in a pill, shot, or nasal spray. Some of the most commonly used hormone drugs for endometriosis are birth control pills, progesterone, danazol, and GnRH agonists.

To prevent a pregnancy, women take birth control pills containing synthetic versions of the hormones estrogen and progesterone. These hormones "fool" your body into thinking that it is already pregnant. They stop the release of hormones that would normally tell your ovaries to release an egg. Taking these pills can slow your period. If you keep taking them without a break, your period will stop. When your period is lighter or doesn't come at all, the endometriosis tissue doesn't grow as much. Also, less menstrual blood flows back through your fallopian tubes. These drugs can help endometriosis, but they do have side effects. They can cause weight gain, bleeding between periods, and sore breasts. They can make you feel nauseated and cause your abdomen to become bloated. If you haven't stopped growing yet, the estrogen in these pills may affect your bones and slow your growth.

Some drugs contain a manufactured form of the hormone progesterone, called progestin. This is one of the same hormones in birth control pills. Progesterone can

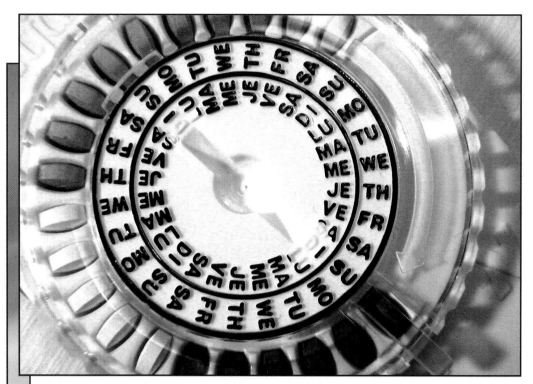

Birth control pills contain synthetic versions of the female hormones estrogen and progesterone. Taking birth control pills can make your period lighter and ease your endometriosis pain.

slow or stop your period. It causes endometriosis tissue to shrink. Side effects include depression, mood swings, bleeding between periods, nausea, and breast soreness.

The synthetic hormone danazol (Danocrine) acts like the male hormone testosterone. Women's bodies make some of this hormone, too. When you take this drug, it stops the release of hormones involved in the menstrual cycle. This prevents ovulation and menstruation. Because it is a male hormone, danazol can cause some unpleasant side effects in girls and women. It can cause you to gain weight. In rare cases, it can increase hair growth on your face and body. It can make your breasts smaller and more tender, and it can give you a deeper voice. Other side effects are acne, mood swings, muscle cramps, tiredness, headaches, dizziness, weakness, and liver problems. Women who take this drug shouldn't get pregnant because it could harm the baby.

Every month, your brain sends a hormone signal to your pituitary gland. The pituitary gland then releases two hormones that tell an ovary to develop and release an egg. Drugs called GnRH agonists do two things: they first make the pituitary gland release more hormones; then they shut down hormone production. This causes the ovaries to stop making estrogen. If you take these drugs, you go into a kind of menopause. Menopause typically happens to older women when their bodies stop making estrogen. It means they permanently stop menstruating and can no longer have babies. Not ovulating or getting a period makes the endometriosis tissue stop growing. Going into a fake menopause can also ease some of your symptoms because you are not menstruating. According to a 2004 report by the National Institutes of Health, the symptoms of endometriosis decrease for many women after menopause because the lesions slowly get smaller. But for some women, the symptoms do not lessen or go away.

GnRH agonists won't stop your symptoms forever, though. As soon as you stop taking them, the symptoms may come back. Also, you can't have a baby while you are on these drugs because you aren't ovulating. Most doctors give their patients these drugs for just six months. Then patients switch treatments or take a break. Side effects of GnRH agonists are like the effects of menopause: hot flashes, night sweats, headaches, depression, loss of bone strength, and vaginal dryness.

Doctors are testing new medicines that work better and have fewer side effects. One is called a GnRH antagonist. It works a lot like GnRH agonists, but it is quicker in stopping the pituitary gland from sending out hormones. Other new drugs can act like estrogen or progesterone in certain parts of the body, but then block these hormones in other parts of the body. Some researchers believe that these drugs slow or stop endometriosis just like birth control pills do, but with fewer side effects. Another new medicine cuts off the blood vessels that feed the problematic endometrial tissue. Without a blood supply, the tissue dies.

SURGERY

If you have a lot of pain or other treatments don't work, your doctor may suggest surgery. For some people, surgery, if it is performed by a doctor who specializes in endometriosis, works better than drugs to treat the disease. But, again, it is not a cure. The condition can come back. Two different kinds of surgery are used to treat endometriosis: laparoscopy and laparotomy.

Laparoscopy

This is the same surgery used to test for endometriosis, as described previously in the tests section. Your doctor can see if you have it and remove tissue at the same time. Taking out the tissue may help relieve your symptoms. The doctor will usually make two cuts, one through which to insert the scope and the other through which to remove the tissue. The cuts made aren't very deep, so you can heal better and more quickly afterward. The doctor will use a thin, lighted scope to help her examine your ovaries, fallopian tubes, uterus, and other organs for lesions.

Your doctor can remove the tissue in one of three ways. She can cut it out with a knife called a scalpel. She can burn it off with high heat from a laser or electrical current. Or, she can destroy it with high-energy sound waves using an ultrasound scalpel. Any surgery has a risk of infection and bleeding. This surgery uses really small cuts, though, so the risks are lower than with major surgery.

Laparotomy

If you have a high stage of endometriosis or the lesions are big, you may need this type of surgery. This surgery may relieve your pain for a longer period of time because it can remove more tissue. It is done through a bigger hole than laparoscopy. The doctor will make an incision in your abdomen to remove the tissue.

If the doctor removes the uterus, it is called a hysterectomy. Depending on where the endometriosis is, the doctor may have to take out the ovaries and fallopian tubes as well. This is called a total hysterectomy. Doctors rarely perform a hysterectomy on young women, though. Because women who have a hysterectomy are not able to give birth to children, it is usually done on older women who have already had children or who don't want to have them. A hysterectomy is a last resort. Doctors will try every other kind of treatment first. Removal of your reproductive organs is a decision you and your parents need to make together with your doctor before your doctor performs the surgery.

Even a hysterectomy won't cure endometriosis. The lesions can be in other parts of the body where the surgery cannot be performed. Or, they may come back after surgery.

Any type of surgery can cause bleeding and infection. The risk is higher with laparotomy than with laparoscopy because the cuts are larger. Also, some women get scar tissue that sticks tissues and even organs together. Scar tissue can cause pain.

ALTERNATIVE TREATMENTS

Medicine and surgery aren't the only ways to treat endometriosis. Some people turn to alternative treatments for relief. These are natural remedies that can sometimes ease pain. Here are some common alternative treatments:

- **Acupuncture.** This technique started in China more than 2,000 years ago. It uses very thin needles to stimulate pressure points on the body. According to traditional Chinese medicine, the points are connected to different parts of the body. Acupuncture does not hurt, and it is very safe. Some people say it relaxes them and eases their pain. For other people, it does not help much. A technique called acupressure is like acupuncture, but it uses pressure instead of needles.
- **Biofeedback.** This technique helps you learn to change functions in your body that you normally can't control, such as your breathing, heart rate, and blood pressure. To teach you how to change these functions, sensors connect your body to a machine. The machine tells you when certain things are happening. It can tell you when your heart rate goes up or your breathing gets faster. It can also tell you when your muscles relax or tighten. Over time, you learn how to control those actions on your own.

- **Guided imagery.** Guided imagery involves mind-body techniques in which people use mental images to promote relaxation and wellness. The techniques involve thinking about something positive to help ease your pain. For example, you visualize walking on a beach or your immune system attacking tissue that is causing pain. Also, by thinking positive thoughts, you can relax, relieve stress, help yourself feel better, and ease your pain.

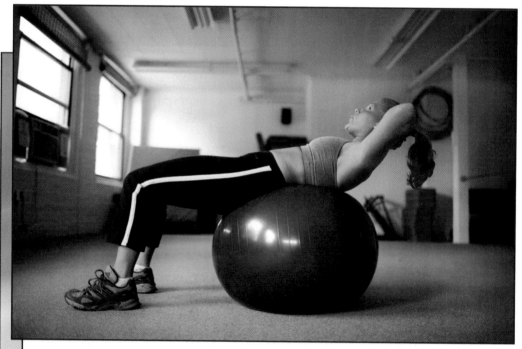

Exercise is one way to help relieve your endometriosis pain. During exercise, the body makes chemicals called endorphins in the brain. Endorphins can help relieve pain in a natural way.

- **Exercise.** Walking, dancing, or doing other types of exercise may help with endometriosis pain. Exercise is good for your body in general. It helps you keep in shape, and it lowers stress.
- **Heat.** A hot bath, shower, or whirlpool bath (such as in a Jacuzzi tub) can be relaxing. Sometimes, heat can relieve pain.
- **Massage.** Research has shown that massage can relax tension in the body. It can soothe sore muscles to reduce pain and relieve stress. You can either visit a licensed massage therapist or ask a friend or family member to rub your back and shoulders.
- **Relaxation.** Stress may make your pain worse. Relaxing with a book or some music can help. Some people find that meditation helps. To meditate, you sit with your eyes closed and control your breathing. You may say a word over and over quietly to help you relax. This word is called a mantra. You can start meditating for just a few minutes at a time and then work up to longer sessions.
- **Yoga.** Some people believe that putting your body into different positions can strengthen your muscles and relieve stress.

It's important to know that some of these alternative treatments can have side effects. You should always check with your doctor before trying any kind of treatment.

Ten Facts About Endometriosis

1. At least 5.5 million women in North America have endometriosis.

2. Endometriosis affects between 2 and 4 percent of women from ages eight to eighty.

3. The prefix "endo-" means "inside," and "metrium" means "womb." Endometriosis occurs when tissue like that in the lining of the uterus is found elsewhere in the body. The uterus is where a pregnant woman carries her unborn baby.

4. Many women wait as long as ten years before being diagnosed with endometriosis.

5. Endometriosis is usually diagnosed in women who are between the ages of twenty-five and thirty-five years old. However, girls younger than eleven and women in their seventies can still have it.

6. In rare cases, lesions can grow as far away from the uterus as the lungs or brain.

7. Infertility affects about 30 to 40 percent of women with endometriosis. But many are able to eventually have children with the help of fertility treatments.

8. Endometrial tissue tends to act the same no matter where it is in the body. Each month it builds up and sheds.

9. The rate of incidence of endometriosis seems to be going up in North America.

10. Some women with endometriosis take birth control pills to stop their periods.

LOOKING TO THE FUTURE

Doctors still don't know what causes endometriosis. They also don't know how to cure it. Doctors want to learn why this tissue grows in some women and not in others. They want to find out if hormones or manufactured chemicals might be partly to blame.

Researchers are also looking at genes, which are instructions that tell cells in our bodies what to do. A mother and father pass genes down to their children. That is why many children look like their parents or get the same diseases their parents have. Researchers are trying to find out which gene, if any, might cause endometriosis. Since every human being has 20,000 or more genes, it's kind of like looking for a needle in a haystack. Researchers are hoping that locating genes related to endometriosis will someday help them understand why certain women get the disease and others do not. They are also hoping that their research will help them find better ways to diagnose and treat the disorder.

Finally, doctors are trying to find new ways to treat endometriosis. They're trying to see if new hormone drugs can help ease pain. One group of drugs is called aromatase inhibitors. These stop the endometriosis tissue from producing the estrogen it needs to grow. Doctors are also looking at drugs that act like estrogen in some tissues, and block the effects of estrogen in other tissues. These types of drugs may work as well as the hormones used

now to treat endometriosis but have fewer side effects.
Also, researchers are looking at alternative treatments
such as acupuncture to relieve pain. Some new treatments
will be available to the public soon. Others may not be
ready for years.

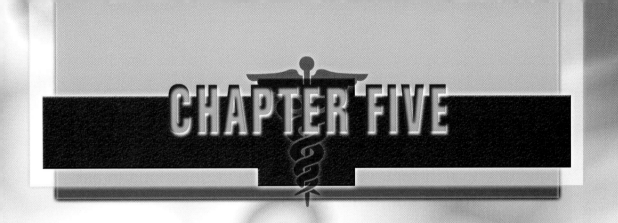

CHAPTER FIVE

What If I Have Endometriosis?

If you have endometriosis, you may feel all alone. You may think that no one in the world understands your pain. You are not alone, though.

If you want to feel better, you first have to take your pain seriously. Don't wait to get help. The earlier you get treatment, the sooner you'll start to feel better. If you feel comfortable doing so, talk to your parents first. Tell them your pain is serious and ask to see a gynecologist.

You may be ashamed to talk with your doctor because this condition affects your reproductive organs. But, remember, doctors are trained to talk about these things. Be honest with your doctor about what you're feeling. If your doctor can't help, ask for a referral to another doctor who knows more about endometriosis. You might want to consider visiting a reproductive endocrinologist who is familiar with treating endometriosis. It is always important to know what your doctor's capabilities are when you choose a specialist to treat your disease.

Ask a lot of questions when you visit your doctor. The more you know about your condition, the more in control you will feel. Here are ten great questions to ask when you're asking for help:

1. Why am I in so much pain?
2. Who is the best doctor(s) to treat me?
3. How can I know for sure whether my symptoms are due to endometriosis?
4. Can I start on medication before I have a pelvic exam and other tests?
5. Will my symptoms get worse if I don't start treatment right away?
6. Are my symptoms bad enough to need surgery or medication?
7. What are the side effects of my treatment?
8. What if treatment won't help my pain?
9. Will I be able to have children some day?
10. Who can I talk to who will help me stop feeling sad about my condition?

Sometimes, it helps to talk to other people who are going through the same experience. These people come together in support groups. There are many endometriosis support groups you can turn to for help. Visit the Endometriosis Association Web site (www.EndometriosisAssn.org) to search for support groups in your state.

Read, Read, Read

You do your homework at school so you can get good grades. Doing your homework when it comes to your health can help you feel better. Read everything you can find on endometriosis. Go to the library and borrow books on the subject. Ask your doctor for pamphlets. Do a search for the word "endometriosis" on the Web.

Learn all about your disease and how it's diagnosed. Find out about the treatments and their side effects. Then you'll know what to expect. You'll also know what questions to ask your doctor. And you'll have good answers ready when your doctor asks you questions.

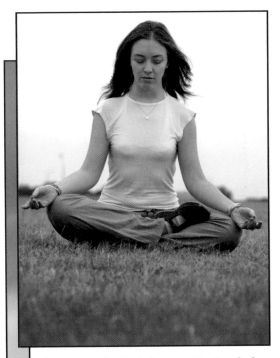

Some people find that meditation helps with endometriosis. To meditate, you focus on your breathing and repeat a word (called a mantra) over and over in your mind to help you relax.

COPING WITH THE PAIN

Endometriosis can be very painful. The pain can be so bad that you can't get out of bed. It can be so bad that you have to miss school and your favorite activities. It can be so bad that it affects your whole life.

You don't have to live in pain, though. First, know how much of it you can handle. Don't try to be brave and bear the pain. When it gets to be too much, know that you can get relief. With your doctor's help, try out different types of pain medicine and techniques until you find what works best for you.

Some people find that natural techniques work. You might try meditation or biofeedback. These methods can relax you and lower stress, which can reduce pain. Exercise is also good for easing pain and stress, and it can make you feel better about your body.

If these techniques work, you may not need anything more. If they don't, you may need over-the-counter pain relievers such as NSAIDs, aspirin, or Tylenol. Or, you may need your doctor to prescribe something stronger. Just be careful if you do take strong painkillers. They can be addictive if you don't use them as your doctor prescribed.

HEALTHY EATING

Medicine is not the only way to heal your body. You also have to take care of it by eating right and exercising. If you feel up to it, exercise at least three days every week. You can take aerobics, dance, do karate, or just walk. Listen to your body, though. You should never feel pain while exercising. If you are ever in pain, stop right away.

It's also important to watch your diet. What you eat can really affect how you feel. Certain foods are better than others for girls and women with endometriosis. Here are some ideas on how to improve your diet:

- **Limit fats.** Fat cells make the hormone estrogen. Endometriosis needs estrogen to grow. A low-fat diet may help control your estrogen level, which might ease your symptoms.

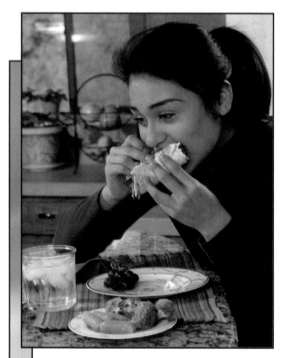

Eating right is an important part of endometriosis treatment. Eat lots of fresh fruits and vegetables, and limit fats and sugars to keep your body as healthy as possible.

- **Cut down on sugar.** You don't have to cut out the hot-fudge sundaes totally; just limit them to once in a while. People with endometriosis are more likely to get a type of yeast infection that harms the immune system. Sugar can make yeast infections worse.

- **Eat plenty of fresh fruits and veggies.** These foods are both low in fat and good for your body.

DEALING WITH YOUR EMOTIONS

You may be experiencing a lot of emotions right now. Those with endometriosis can feel afraid, angry, ashamed, and stressed out. Don't take out your emotions on family and friends. Yelling at the people who care about you can cause you even more stress and strain.

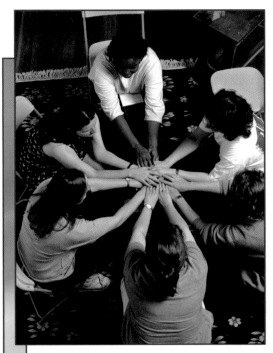

A support group can help you see that you are not the only one with endometriosis. Talking to other people who have the same disease can help you feel better about what you're going through, learn from others' experiences and treatments, and find new strategies for coping with your endometriosis.

Simply talking to others can help you feel better. You may feel most comfortable talking to your parents or other family members, especially those who have some experience with endometriosis. Or, you might prefer to talk to your friends or teachers. The people who care about you will want to help you through this. Listening is just one way they can give support. Offering to do your chores or help with your homework are other ways.

If it's not you, but your friend, sister, or

mother who has endometriosis, be available to listen. That is the most important thing you can do. Take what she's feeling seriously. If she is feeling very depressed or angry, encourage her to get help.

Sometimes, it helps to see a counselor who is experienced in dealing with health problems to talk through your feelings. Counselors are trained to help people deal with their emotions. You may find that talking about your problems with an expert or members of a support group will enable you to cope better.

Your pain and embarrassment may make you feel like curling up in your room alone. But it's important for you to get out and keep doing the things you love. Having fun will keep your spirits up. When your mind is happy, your body tends to feel better, too.

Above all, keep a positive attitude. Don't give up. Know that you can get relief from your symptoms. Many people with endometriosis lead very active, happy lives.

GLOSSARY

computed tomography (CT) An X-ray scanning technique that makes detailed, three-dimensional images of your internal organs and outer body. A computer combines the scans into images.

contraception Prevention of pregnancy.

embryo A human in the early stages of fetal growth, from conception to the eighth week of pregnancy.

endometriosis A disease that occurs when tissue like that of the lining of the uterus grows in other parts of the body. The immune system does not act correctly in response to this disease.

endometrium Tissue that lines the inside of the uterus and builds up and sheds each month during the menstrual cycle.

fetus An unborn human from the eighth week of pregnancy until birth.

gynecologist A doctor who specializes in women's sexual and reproductive health, including breast care, menstrual health, and birth control.

hormones Chemicals released by the body that tell other parts of the body what to do.

hysterectomy Surgery to remove the uterus. Sometimes, the doctor will take out the fallopian tubes and ovaries, too. Women who have this surgery will not be able to have children.

infertility The condition of not being able to have a child, or having trouble conceiving or carrying a pregnancy to full term.

in vitro fertilization Mixing sperm from the man and an egg from the woman to make an embryo in a lab.

laparoscopy A test that uses a thin, lighted scope to look inside the abdomen. Sometimes, the procedure includes taking out endometriosis tissue.

laparotomy Surgery to remove endometriosis tissue.

lymph vessels Tubes that carry a fluid called lymph around the body. Lymph contains fluid and cells that fight infection.

magnetic resonance imaging (MRI) A technique that uses magnets and radio waves to take pictures of the inner body.

menopause When a woman's periods stop. This usually happens at around the age of fifty.

menstrual cycle The monthly reproductive cycle in a woman's body. An egg matures, is released, and the uterine lining sheds if the egg is not fertilized by sperm.

ovulation The release of a mature egg from the ovary.

prostaglandins Substances that are similar to hormones and that affect pain and inflammation.

ultrasound A procedure that uses high-energy sound waves to look inside the body.

FOR MORE INFORMATION

Canadian Women's Health Network
419 Graham Avenue, Suite 203
Winnipeg, MB R3C 0M3
Canada
(204) 942-5500
Web site: http://www.cwhn.ca
This group offers education and support for many women's
health issues.

Endometriosis Association
International Headquarters
8585 N. 76th Place
Milwaukee, WI 53223
(800) 992-3636 (U.S. and Canada)
(414) 355-2200
Web site: http://www.EndometriosisAssn.org
The Endometriosis Association has hundreds of support
groups worldwide and conducts research in six countries.
It has a teen newsletter and a mentor program that teams
a teen with another woman who has endometriosis who
can be helpful in sharing experiences with endometriosis.

International Pelvic Pain Society
Women's Medical Plaza, Suite 402
2006 Brookwood Medical Center Drive
Birmingham, AL 35209
(205) 877-2950
Web site: http://www.pelvicpain.org
This society aims to improve quality of life for anyone
with pelvic pain.

National Women's Health Network
514 10th Street NW, Suite 400
Washington, DC 20004
(202) 628-7814
Web site: http://www.nwhn.org
This group is a voice for all types of women's health issues.

WEB SITES

Due to the changing nature of Internet links, the Rosen
Publishing Group, Inc., has developed an online list of
Web sites related to the subject of this book. This site is
updated regularly. Please use this link to access the list:

http://www.rosenlinks.com/lsh/endo

FOR FURTHER READING

Ballweg, Mary Lou. *Endometriosis: The Complete Reference for Taking Charge of Your Health*. New York, NY: McGraw-Hill, 2004.

Ballweg, Mary Lou. *The Endometriosis Sourcebook*. Chicago, IL: Contemporary Books, 1995.

Cassan, Adolpho. *The Reproductive System*. Philadelphia, PA: Chelsea Clubhouse, 2005.

Gravelle, Karen, and Jennifer Gravelle. *The Period Book: Everything You Don't Want to Ask (But Need to Know)*. Illustrated by Debbie Palen. New York, NY: Walker Books for Young Readers, 1996.

Henderson, Lorraine, and Ros Wood. *Explaining Endometriosis*. New South Wales, Australia: Allen & Unwin, 2001.

Loulan, JoAnn, and Bonnie Worthen. *Period: A Girl's Guide to Menstruation with a Parent's Guide*. Minnetonka, MN: Book Peddlers, 2001.

Lyons, Thomas, and Cheryl Kimball. *What to Do When the Doctor Says It's Endometriosis*. Gloucester, MA: Fair Winds Press, 2003.

Parker, Steve. *The Reproductive System: Injury, Illness and Health*. Chicago, IL: Heinemann Library, 2004.

BIBLIOGRAPHY

Allen, C., S. Hopewell, and A. Prentice. "Non-steroidal Anti-inflammatory Drugs for Pain in Women with Endometriosis." *Cochrane Database of Systematic Reviews*, October 19, 2005.

Ballweg, Mary Lou. *Endometriosis: The Complete Reference for Taking Charge of Your Health*. New York, NY: McGraw-Hill, 2004.

BBC News. "Endometriosis Cancer Risk." Retrieved March 2, 2006 (http://news.bbc.co.uk/1/hi/health/3045938.stm).

Canavan, Timothy P., and Lee Radosh. "Managing Endometriosis: Strategies to Minimize Pain and Damage." *Postgraduate Medicine*, March 2000, pp. 213–224.

The Cleveland Clinic. "Surgical Treatment for Endometriosis." Retrieved October 30, 2005 (http://www.clevelandclinic.org/health/health-info/docs/0300/0338.asp?index=4620).

Endometriosis Research Center. "Think 'Killer Cramps' Are Normal? Think Again!" Retrieved October 30, 2005 (http://www.endocenter.org/killercramps.htm).

Fromer, Margot Joan. *The Endometriosis Survival Guide*. Oakland, CA: New Harbinger Publications, 1998.

Gupta, Janesh, and Rajesh Varma. "The Latest Thinking on Endometriosis." *Pulse*, January 29, 2005, p. 48.

Johnson, Ellen T. "Your Initial Endometriosis Appointment: Questions the Doctor May Ask You." Retrieved December 3, 2005 (http://www.endozone.org/display.asp?page = endometriosis-coping-zone_0303_initial-endometriosis-appointment).

The Merck Manual of Medical Information. "Endometriosis." Retrieved October 30, 2005 (http://www.merck.com/mmhe/sec22/ch245/ch245a.html).

National Institute of Child Health and Human Development. "Endometriosis." Retrieved October 30, 2005 (http://www.nichd.nih.gov/publications/pubs/endometriosis/index.htm).

National Women's Health Information Center. "Frequently Asked Questions About Endometriosis." December 2002. Retrieved October 30, 2005 (http://www.4woman.gov/faq/endomet.pdf).

Nemours Foundation. "Endometriosis." kidshealth.org. Updated September 2004. Retrieved October 30, 2005 (http://www.kidshealth.org/teen/sexual_health/girls/endometriosis.html).

NewMyer, Kristi. "Endometriosis." Retrieved December 3, 2005 (http://altmed.creighton.edu/endometriosis/about_endometriosis.htm).

Wilson, Amanda. "Endometriosis: A Common Cause of Infertility and Pelvic Pain." *Journal of the American Academy of Physician Assistants*, December 2003, pp. 20–23.

INDEX

C

cancer, 26–27

E

endometriosis
    described, 5, 8–9, 23
    diagnosing, 27, 30–32, 49
    discovery of, 15–17
    myths and facts about, 20
    stages of, 32–34
    statistics on, 5, 19, 25, 46
    symptoms of, 5, 9, 14, 23–25
    testing for, 30
    theories on cause of, 15–19, 47
    treatments for, 22, 30–31, 32,
        35–48, 52
exercise, 21, 45, 52

F

female reproductive system, 9–12

G

gynecologist, first visit to, 27–30

H

Halban, Joseph, 17

I

infertility, 25–26, 46

L

laparoscopy, 10, 31–32, 41, 42

M

menopause, 39–40
menstruation
    cramps/pain and, 5, 20
    described, 9, 11, 12–14
    hormones and, 37, 38, 39
    start of, 4, 19
Meyer, R., 17–18

N

nutrition, 21, 52–53

O

ovarian cysts, 25
ovulation, 12, 37, 39, 40

P

pregnancy, 12, 13, 25, 26, 37, 39
prostaglandins, 23

S

Sampson, John, 15–17
support groups, 50, 55

V

von Rokitansky, Karl, 15

ABOUT THE AUTHOR

Stephanie Watson is a writer and editor based in Atlanta, Georgia. She has written or contributed to more than a dozen health and science books, including *Encyclopedia of the Human Body: The Endocrine System*, *The Mechanisms of Genetics: An Anthology of Current Thought*, and *Science and Its Times*. Ms. Watson is also executive editor of *Focus on Healthy Aging*, a national monthly publication.

PHOTO CREDITS

Cover, p. 4 © www.istockphoto.com/ericsphotography; cover, pp. 1, 4 (silhouette) © www.istockphoto.com/jamesbenet; p. 1 (inset) CDC/ Dr. Edwin P. Ewing, Jr.; p. 6 © www.istockphoto.com/Oleg Prikhodko; p. 9 © Véronique Estiot/Photo Researchers, Inc.; p. 11 © Wainwright/ Custom Medical Stock Photo; p. 13 © Clouds Hill Imaging Ltd./Corbis; p. 16 © John Bavosi/Photo Researchers, Inc.; p. 18 © Joseph Sohm, ChromoSohm Inc./Corbis; p. 21 © www.istockphoto.com/Galina Barskaya; p. 24 © VEM/Photo Researchers, Inc.; p. 29 © Ronnie Kaufman/ Corbis; p. 31 © Nicolas Edwige/Photo Researchers, Inc.; p. 33 Fertility Institute of the Mid-South and Dan Martin MD, Memphis; p. 36 © Mario Tama/Getty Images; p. 38 © www.istockphoto.com/Allison Marles; p. 44 © Steve Prezant/Corbis; p. 51 © www.istockphoto.com/Andresr; pp. 53, 54 © Bob Daemmrich/The Image Works; back cover (top to bottom) CDC/Dr. E. Arum, Dr. N. Jacobs, CDC/Dr. Edwin P. Ewing, Jr., CDC/Joe Miller, CDC/Joe Miller, CDC/Dr. Edwin P. Ewing, Jr., CDC.

Designer: Nelson Sá; **Editor:** Kathy Kuhtz Campbell
Photo Researcher: Amy Feinberg